# The Pregnant Parent's Guide to Newborn Care

# Table of Contents

# Chapter 1. Introduction

Welcoming a new life into the world is as thrilling as it is fulfilling, but it can also raise a myriad of questions and concerns. In our special report on "The Pregnant Parent's Guide to Newborn Care," we delve deep into the magical journey right from the golden hour after birth through the ensuing months of uncharted waters. Aimed at alleviating your anxieties and building a strong foundation, this comprehensive but easy-to-understand guide shines a light on newborn care, crucial milestones, health indicators, and nurturing techniques. It's the ultimate roadmap for the greatest adventure of your life, making this journey less about surviving and more about enjoying your early days with your infant. Our report doesn't only dispense wisdom; it builds confidence, turning apprehensive parents-to-be into knowledgeable care-givers ready to embrace parenthood fully. Engaging, practical and peppered with a dose of encouragement, it's an indispensable resource you wouldn't want to miss! So buckle in, your beautiful journey of love, joy and discovery is about to get a whole lot easier, one page at a time. Let's embark on this beautiful journey together!

# Chapter 2. The Magic of the Golden Hour

The moment your newborn enters the world, a special clock starts ticking – the hour following birth, often referred to as the 'golden hour,' heralds a unique time of bonding and vital health-checks. This magical period, filled with firsts and potent experiences, sets the groundwork for the parent-infant bond and newborn health.

## 2.1. The First Embrace

The very first aspect of the golden hour is immediate skin-to-skin contact. This should ideally take place within the first few minutes after birth. The baby is dried, and then placed belly-down on one of the parent's bare chest, typically the mother. A warm blanket is put over the baby, and this intimate contact is maintained.

This skin-to-skin contact manifests numerous benefits. For one, it helps regulate the baby's temperature more effectively than an incubator. It stabilizes the baby's heart rate, breathing pattern, and helps improve the oxygen saturation levels. Plus, it stimulates digestion and an interest in feeding.

Moreover, it encourages the release of a hormone called oxytocin, often referred to as the 'bonding hormone.' This hormone promotes attachment, relaxes mother and baby, and has a host of health benefits for both. In this peaceful time, most babies will begin searching for the breast and attempt to breastfeed.

## 2.2. Initial Breastfeeding

Breastfeeding in the golden hour initiates the process of lactation in the mother. It aids in uterine contraction, which in turn helps in reducing the risk of postpartum hemorrhage. Also, the first milk, colostrum, a substance that is yellow to orange in color and thick and sticky, is filled with high-duty nutrients and antibodies. It's an optimal first food for the baby.

Colostrum, the baby's first vaccine, has a laxative effect and aids in the expulsion of the baby's first stool, called meconium. This helps minimize bilirubin levels and reduces the risk of jaundice. The act of sucking on the breast also improves coordination between breathing and swallowing.

# 2.3. Medical Checks in the Golden Hour

In addition to immediate bonding and first feeding, several practical and necessary assessments and interventions typically take place during the golden hour. These help ensure the baby's safe transition to life outside the womb.

One essential check is the Apgar score, assessed at one and five minutes after birth. The Apgar test checks the baby's Heart Rate, Muscle Tone, Reflex Response, Color, and Respiration - the initials leading to the mnemonic APGAR.

Although the golden hour is a sacred time, certain medical interventions beneficial to the newborn's well-being are recommended:

1. Vitamin K injection: Newborns are born with low levels of vitamin K, a vital component in helping the blood clot. An injection of Vitamin K can prevent a rare but life-threatening condition known as 'vitamin K deficiency bleeding' or VKDB.

2. Application of a topical antibiotic ointment to the baby's eyes: This prevents neonatal conjunctivitis due to STIs like gonorrhea and chlamydia.

3. Newborn screening and metabolic tests: These diagnostic tests can identify certain genetic, metabolic, hormonal and functional conditions.

## 2.4. Conclusion

The golden hour is the first chapter in a parent's journey, and understanding its significance is of prime importance. It is indeed a magical time, teeming with powerful milestones, pivotal to the well-being of the newborn and the bonding process between newborn and parents.

Staying informed is crucial for expectant parents as they navigate this magical 'golden' time. The golden hour presents a mesmerizing, once-in-a-lifetime moment, that initiates the bond of love and dependence that plays an immense role in the infant's growth and development. Embrace these sixty minutes and cherish them. Begin your journey of parenthood on a note of love, care, and confidence - they will guide you and your baby onto a path of health and happiness.

# Chapter 3. Understanding Newborn Health Indicators

Welcoming a newborn into your life can bring about a flurry of emotions and uncertainties, particularly about recognizing and interpreting their health indicators. Owning knowledge of these indicators is a vital part of your journey as a parent.

## 3.1. Understanding Newborn Skin

A newborn's skin can tell a lot about their health status. At birth, babies often have a whitish, waxy coating known as vernix, which gradually disappears a few days after birth. It's common to see changes in your newborn's skin color due to temperature changes, crying, or certain medical conditions.

A bluish color in hands and feet, also known as acrocyanosis, is quite common within the first few days after birth and usually isn't a cause for concern. However, a blue color in the face, lips, or torso needs an immediate medical attention as it may denote inadequate oxygen supply.

Jaundice, characterized by yellowing of the skin and whites of the eyes, typically appears two to four days after birth, affecting almost 60% of all newborns. Mild jaundice is usually harmless, but if it persists, medical evaluation becomes necessary.

Baby acne, a result of maternal hormones, can appear within the first month and usually clears up on its own. A rash of tiny, red spots, known as erythema toxicum, may also appear on your baby's face, chest, and back, which is harmless and will disappear within a week.

# 3.2. Decoding Newborn Behavior

Newborns communicate through behavior patterns. Observing your baby's sleep and wakefulness cycles, feeding cues and patterns, body movements, gaze directions, various cries, and facial expressions can help decode their wants and needs.

Most newborns sleep an average of 16-17 hours a day, spending more time in REM sleep than adults which is essential for their brain development. They wouldn't stick to a schedule for the initial few weeks. Over time, their sleep schedules start to consolidate to longer periods.

Your baby is likely hungry if they put their hands to their mouth, make sucking noises, move their mouth when you touch their cheek, or fuss. Crying is a late sign of hunger, and awaiting it could lead your baby to lose energy, making feeding more challenging.

# 3.3. Newborn Physical Indicators

Maintaining a regular check-up schedule will help your pediatrician track your baby's physical growth and development.

The average newborn weight is around 7.5 lbs (3.4 kg), and it's normal for newborns to lose weight during the initial days after birth. But they usually regain their birth weight by about 10-14 days of age. Babies typically grow 1.5 to 2.5 cm per month and gain daily 25-30 grams (5-7 ounces per week) in the first six months.

Checking your newborn's soft spots, or fontanels, is another important health indicator. These areas aid in your baby's brain growth and typically close by 18 months. A sunken fontanel can be a sign of dehydration, while a bulging one might suggest increased pressure on the brain and should be evaluated by a healthcare provider.

# 3.4. Understanding Newborn Reflexes

Newborn reflexes are automatic responses to particular stimuli, which gives insight into the infant's nervous system and development. Here are a few essential ones.

1. Rooting Reflex: When stroked or touched on the cheek, your newborn will turn their head and open their mouth to root in the direction of the touch. This reflex helps them find the breast or bottle to feed.

2. Sucking Reflex: When the roof of a baby's mouth is touched, they will start to suck.

3. Grasp Reflex: Stroke the palm of your baby's hand and you'll notice the fingers closing as if grasping. Similarly, if you stroke the bottom of their foot, their toes will curl downward.

4. Moro or Startle Reflex: When your baby is startled by a loud sound or movement, they may react by stretching out their arms and legs, arching their back, and then pulling them back in.

5. Stepping Reflex: When held upright with their feet touching a flat surface, your baby will appear to take steps or dance. This doesn't mean they're ready to walk, but it does indicate normal limb movement and coordination.

Thumb rule is that all these reflexes disappear as the baby grows, giving way to more voluntary control over movements.

This comprehensive, yet easy-to-understand guide on newborn health indicators is a stepping stone to becoming more confident parents. As you navigate through this rewarding journey, always remember to seek advice from healthcare professionals for any concerns. The voyage may seem challenging, rest assured, with knowledge and guidance, you and your baby will sail through it with grace and joy.

# Chapter 4. Mastering Diapering and Bath Time Basics

The first step to mastering diapering is acquiring the necessary gear: a changing table or clean, soft surface; a supply of disposable or cloth diapers; fasteners if you're using cloth diapers; diaper ointment; and wipes or a couple of damp, clean cloths for cleaning your baby's bottom.

Consider keeping a handy diaper toolkit stocked with wipes, fresh diapers, and rash cream within your reach whenever you're changing diapers, to ensure you have all the essentials at your fingertips. It's also wise to have a spare change of clothing for your baby close by, in case they need a quick change after a particularly messy diaper.

## 4.1. The Diaper Changing Process

Begin by laying your baby down on the changing table or surface. Always keep one hand on your baby; the safety strap found on most changing tables is not enough to thoroughly secure an active, wriggling baby. Using your free hand, open a clean diaper and put it within easy reach.

Next, unfasten the dirty diaper but leave it under your infant. Using the front half of the diaper, wipe your baby's bottom clean. For a baby girl, always wipe from front to back to prevent infections. Remove any remaining debris with wipes or damp cloths, again wiping from front to back for a girl.

Once the baby is clean, remove the dirty diaper and set it out for disposal. At this point, if you see any signs of diaper rash, apply diaper ointment before proceeding.

Finally, lift your baby gently by the ankles and slide a clean diaper underneath them. The back part with the adhesive strips should go under your baby's bottom. Bring the front part up over your baby's belly. For a boy, ensure that he's pointing downwards so that he doesn't urinate out of the top of the diaper. Fasten the diaper at both sides with the adhesive strips, ensuring it's snug but not so tight that it impedes movement or cuts into your baby's skin.

## 4.2. Tips for Diapering

There are a few general rules to remember when diapering an infant.

Always wash your hands before and after every diaper change. This promotes cleanliness and significantly reduces the chance of spreading germs. If you're on the go, use a hand sanitizer.

During the newborn stage, babies often need changing as frequently as every 2-3 hours, around ten times a day. However, this slows down as the baby grows older.

You'll know your baby needs a change if they seem uncomfortable or restless, or if the diaper feels full. Most of the new-age diapers have a color-changing wetness indicator function that displays a blue line when it's time for a change.

Remember to check your baby's diaper regularly, especially overnight. Babies often wake from sleep because they need changing, so a dry diaper might mean a little more sleep for you too!

## 4.3. Bath Time Basics

Bathing your newborn can be a tender bonding experience but can also seem daunting for first-time parents. Keep in mind; newborns only require a bath 2 to 3 times a week. More frequent bathing might dry their skin.

Before you begin, gather your bathing essentials: a baby bathtub or a spare sink, a couple of towels (one for washing, one for drying), mild baby soap, a clean diaper, and fresh clothes.

## 4.4. The Bathing Process

Start by filling the tub or sink with around 2inches of warm water. The water temperature should be checked with your wrist or elbow, and it should feel warm, not hot. Undress your newborn, wrap them in a towel, and then slowly slip them into the tub, feet first, using one hand to support their neck and head. Once they're comfortably in, you can start bathing them.

Washing should be done from top to bottom. Begin by gently splashing some warm water on your baby's body to keep them warm. Use a soft baby cloth or your hand to clean their face. Be careful to avoid the area around their eyes. Then, using a minimal amount of soap, wash your baby's body from the neck down. Don't forget the creases under the arms, behind the ears, around the neck, and in the diaper area.

To clean the head, gently massage a bit of soap into the hair and scalp. You can then rinse this off along with the soap from the body, using your free hand to shield your baby's eyes.

Once you've rinsed the soap off, gently lift your baby out of the tub, using one hand to support their neck and head. Immediately wrap them in a dry towel and pat them dry, again bearing in mind areas like underarms, behind ears, and the diaper area. Avoid vigorous rubbing as this can irritate your baby's skin.

Now, with your baby clean and dry, it's time for a fresh diaper and clean clothes. Remember, this activity should be calm and soothing.

You may choose to follow the bath with a gentle massage, which can help relax your baby and prepare them for sleep.

# 4.5. Tips for Bathing

Never leave your infant unattended in water, even for a second. Infants can easily slip or roll into the water and can drown in even just an inch or two.

Newborns can quickly get cold, so ensure the room is warm, free of drafts, and that bath water maintains an appropriate temperature throughout the bath.

Use only products designed specifically for babies. They should be gentle, hypoallergenic, and free of dyes, parabens, and fragrances.

Remember, mastering diapering and bathing basics is not just about the process, but also developing a recurring routine that both you and your baby find soothing and comfortable. With time, patience, and lots of practice, it will soon become second nature to you.

Remember to enjoy these moments as you nurture and bond with your baby during these early months. They pass only too quickly!

# Chapter 5. Feeding Fundamentals: Breastfeeding and Formula

Feeding your newborn is one of the first tasks you perform as a new parent, and it's a special bonding moment. Whether you breastfeed or use formula, it is crucial to understand the mechanics, benefits, and potential challenges of both feeding methods.

## 5.1. The Basics of Breastfeeding

Breastfeeding is a natural process where a mother feeds her baby with breast milk, which is produced in her milk ducts after childbirth. While breastfeeding may come naturally for some, it can take patience, practice, and support for many others.

First, it's essential to ensure that your baby latches onto your breast correctly. Bring your baby's mouth to your nipple, ensuring their lips are on the much larger, darker part of your breast, the areola. The correct latch can make the difference between a comfortable and painful breastfeeding experience.

Breastfeeding is recommended by most health organizations as it offers numerous benefits to both mother and baby. Let's delve into them.

## 5.2. Benefits of Breastfeeding

Breast milk is an excellent nutrition source for your newborn because it contains the right balance of nutrients necessary for growth and development. Not only that, but it also changes as your baby grows, meeting their evolving nutritional needs.

1. **Immune Boost**: Breast milk is packed with antibodies that can't be engineered. They protect your baby from numerous infections and diseases.

2. **Lower SIDS Risk**: Breastfeeding may lower your baby's risk of Sudden Infant Death Syndrome (SIDS).

3. **Enhanced Bonding**: The skin-to-skin contact during breastfeeding can help develop a closer bond between you and your baby.

For mothers, breastfeeding helps the body recover from childbirth faster, reduces the risk of certain cancers, and even aids in weight loss after delivery.

Despite its unparalleled benefits, breastfeeding may not always be possible or enough for some infants. In such cases, formula feeding becomes a viable and nutritious option.

# 5.3. The Basics of Formula Feeding

Infant formula is a manufactured food designed to feed babies under 12 months old. It is usually based on cow's milk but is modified to resemble breast milk as closely as possible, providing all the necessary nutrients an infant needs for growth and development.

When preparing a bottle of formula, you need to measure the right amount of formula and warm water. Make sure to follow the instructions on the formula package closely. Shake the bottle to mix the formula, then test a drop on your wrist to ensure it's not too hot. During feeding, hold your baby slightly upright and hold the bottle to their lips.

# 5.4. Benefits of Formula Feeding

While it doesn't offer the same composition as breast milk, formula has its own advantages.

1. **Convenience**: Parents can share feeding duties, allowing mothers to rest or return to work.

2. **Flexible Timing**: Unlike breast milk, which needs constant feeding or pumping, formula-fed babies can go slightly longer between feedings.

3. **Dietary Freedom**: Mothers who formula feed don't need to worry about their own diet affecting their babies.

Deciding the best way to feed your baby is a personal decision. It's entirely possible to combine both breastfeeding and formula-feeding based on what works best for your family.

# 5.5. Dealing with Common Feeding Concerns

In the journey of engaging in feeding, both breastfeeding and formula, new parents often face a range of common feeding concerns. Let's address a few.

1. **Low Milk Supply**: If you're breastfeeding and feel you have low milk supply, feed your baby frequently and remove milk from your breast often. If the problem persists, consult a lactation consultant.

2. **Latching Issues**: Some babies may have trouble latching onto the breast. A lactation consultant can provide expert guidance on different feeding positions.

3. **Digestive Troubles**: If your baby has constipation, excess gas, or diarrhea, they might be intolerant to certain proteins in breast milk or formula. Consult your pediatrician about potential solutions.

Getting off to the right start with feeding will give your baby the best nutrients and foster a deeper bond between you. Remember, every child is different, and what works best for your family is the ultimate feeding choice. You're doing a great job, and you have resources and support around you for any questions or concerns you may face during this important time of nurturing.

# Chapter 6. Decoding Your Newborn's Sleep Patterns

A newborn's world of sleep might seem cryptic and erratic at first, but there is a method to the madness, and patterns do emerge over time. Getting acquainted with these patterns can help you anticipate your baby's sleeping cycles and adjust your own schedules accordingly. This might sound daunting, but rest easy - we're here to decode it all for you.

## 6.1. The Norms of Newborn Sleep

Unlike the structured sleep routines we adults are accustomed to, infants operate on an entirely different schedule. There is no night or day for a newborn, and their sleep patterns are predominantly governed by their hunger cycles. On average, newborns sleep for a staggering total of 14 to 17 hours a day, albeit in shorter bursts of 2 to 4 hours.

Your newborn's sleep cycle is much shorter than an adult's, with each cycle about 50 minutes long, involving periods of REM (rapid eye movement) and non-REM sleep. Newborns are prone to twitching, smiling, or sucking during REM sleep which can consume about half of their total sleep time. Moreover, babies get a majority of their growth hormone – crucial for development – during this sleep phase.

## 6.2. Understanding the Stages of Sleep

To understand your baby's sleep patterns, it's important to comprehend the various stages of sleep which include:

1. Drowsiness: In this stage, the baby's eyes start to droop and they may doze off intermittently. Your baby might look sleepy but might startle or wake up with small disturbances.

2. REM sleep: Babies spend about half of their sleep in this stage, which is distinguished by darting eyes under the eyelids, rapid breath, twitching and restlessness. This is a light stage of sleep where they could easily be awakened.

3. Light non-REM sleep: During this stage, babies may stir and their eyes may flutter open and closed a bit. However, they can still be awakened rather easily.

4. Deep non-REM sleep: Here, your baby lies still and may not show any movement or noise. They become less responsive to noise around them and it becomes a lot harder to wake them up.

Understanding these stages can help parents gauge when not to disturb a baby, which allows for better sleep hygiene and overall health.

# 6.3. The Role of Feeding in Sleep

Newborns primarily sleep, wake, and eat in cycles – with no clear distinction between day and night. In the early weeks, expect your baby to wake up often for feedings. It's recommended that newborns be woken up every 3 to 4 hours if they haven't risen for a feed spontaneously.

Maintaining a feeding diary that tracks how often your baby was fed, for how long and when he slept could be instrumental in identifying patterns and planning your day accordingly.

# 6.4. The Emergence of a Sleep Schedule

Though it may seem like your newborn has no sense of day or night, their internal clock will start to adjust at about 6 weeks. You'll likely notice your baby starting to stay awake more during the day and sleeping for longer spans at night, gradually syncing their sleep schedule with the rest of the family.

It's important to remember that building an effective sleep routine takes time, patience, and consistency. Recognizing your baby's sleep cues, establishing a calming bedtime routine, and creating a sleep-friendly environment can go a long way in fostering healthy sleep habits.

# 6.5. Sleep and Milestone Achievements

While it's tempting to attribute changes in sleep patterns to growth spurts, do remember that changes could also be linked to developmental milestones or even conditions like illness or teething. Be open to interpreting these alterations as signs of your baby's growth and change.

# 6.6. When to Seek Professional Help

Keep an eye out for potential sleep-related problems like regular, notable snoring, long pauses between breaths, extreme difficulty waking the baby up, or disruptions in sleep due to trouble breathing. If you notice any of these issues, it's best to consult your pediatrician promptly.

In sum, understanding your newborn's sleep patterns may seem like a riddle, but with time and keen observation, you'll start to recognize patterns. A newborn's sleep schedule largely depends on their feeding schedule for the first few weeks, and slowly, a sleep pattern will emerge. Being patient, and maintaining a consistent bedtime routine, will surely help foster healthy sleep habits. You're doing fantastic, and we're here to help you navigate this journey! Your newborn may not thank you now, but the sleep manners you help them cultivate will serve them well in their years ahead!

# Chapter 7. Managing Common Health Concerns

Whether during the wee hours of the night or in the bustling brightness of the day, as a new parent, you might find yourself dealing with common health concerns regarding your newborn. Knowledge and preparedness lay the foundation for nurturing your baby confidently and effectively. This comprehensive discussion is aimed at imparting you with insights about managing the common health concerns your infant might encounter.

## 7.1. Newborn Skin Conditions

Understanding your baby's skin is crucial as it serves as a compelling indicator of their health status. Don't be startled if your baby's skin isn't as perfect as you imagined as newborn skin is sensitive and can exhibit a variety of conditions.

- *Baby Acne:* This condition appears at 2 to 3 weeks of age. Small red or white bumps on your baby's cheeks, nose, and forehead are common symptoms. In most cases, baby acne disappears on its own within a few months. However, if it persists beyond a few months, kindly seek pediatric consultation.

- *Cradle Cap:* The presence of rough, scaly patches on your baby's scalp symbolize Cradle Cap. Regular shampooing and brushing can aid in reducing them. Again, if they last longer, your pediatrician can recommend a suitable medicated shampoo.

Remember, normal newborn skin is thin, less hairy, and less sweaty, hence it requires gentle care. Limiting bath time and using hypoallergenic products can be beneficial for your baby's skin health.

# 7.2. Feeding and Digestive Health Problems

Feeding and digestion-related issues are quite common in newborns. If your baby appears uncomfortable during or after feeding, they might face underlying digestive problems.

- *Reflux:* Babies often spit up milk due to immature gastrointestinal tracts. However, if the baby is not gaining weight due to excessive spit up or vomit, medical attention is required.

- *Constipation:* If your baby appears uncomfortable during bowel movements or passes hard stool, they may be constipated. Pediatric-approved remedies such as a small amount of water or apple juice may help. Persistent constipation needs immediate attention.

Remember that feeding positions matter. Hold your baby upright during feeding times and for at least 30 minutes afterwards to prevent digestive issues.

# 7.3. Common Infant Diseases

Babies are vulnerable to infections and diseases due to their developing immune system. Recognizing signs early can help manage these effectively.

- *Cold:* Symptoms include stuffy or runny nose and mild fever. Keeping your baby hydrated and suctioning out nasal passages can provide relief. If symptoms last more than a week or escalate, seek medical attention.

- *Thrush:* It is a type of yeast infection that presents as white patches in your baby's mouth or tongue that resemble cottage cheese. If your baby refuses feedings or is uncomfortable, contact a healthcare professional for suitable treatment.

Vaccination plays an essential role in preventing severe infections and diseases. Keeping your baby's vaccination schedule up to date is of utmost importance.

## 7.4. Sleep-related Concerns

Newborns sleep a lot but in short bursts. Ensuring that your baby gets adequate sleep aids in their growth and development.

- *Night-Day sleep reversal:* Babies often mix up day and night. You can help by limiting daytime naps and keeping nights quiet. With time, babies usually figure out the right time to sleep.

- *Sleep-Related Breathing Issues:* If your baby snorts, gasps, or has long pauses in their breathing while sleeping, it could indicate sleep apnea. It is a severe condition that needs medical intervention.

Good sleeping habits from an early age ensure healthy growth and development. Always put your baby to sleep on their back to minimize the risk of Sudden Infant Death Syndrome (SIDS).

The health concerns mentioned here are commonplace but not exhaustive. A baby's health can change rapidly, and as parents, your instincts hold great value. Trust your instincts and seek help if needed. Regular pediatric check-ups aid in early detection and management of potential health issues, bolstering your baby's progression into a healthy and happy being. Lastly, always remember that it's okay to ask for help - you are not alone in this parenthood journey.

# Chapter 8. Adapting to Developmental Milestones

The early months of parenthood are characterized by a whirlwind of change, nurturing, and constant learning. It is during this time that you will begin to understand your baby's developmental milestones—specific physical and behavioral markers that serve as checkpoints in your child's progress.

## 8.1. The First Month: Shifting from Reflexive to Controlled Movements

Infants in their first month of life primarily exhibit reflexive movements. However, some developmental strides take place even during this very early period.

- Physical development: Newborns can lift their heads momentarily during tummy time and will reflexively clutch anything that touches their palm or foot—a phenomenon known as the grasp reflex. Your baby's movements might appear jerky or spasmodic, but it's all a part of their developing control over their body.

- Social and emotional development: Your baby will start recognizing the voice and smell of the primary caregiver. Even though their vision is still quite blurry, they enjoy looking at contrasts and faces positioned 8 to 12 inches away.

- Cognitive development: Babies express their needs through crying. It's essential to respond and comfort them promptly to foster feelings of security and trust.

## 8.2. Second to the Fourth Month: Developing Intentions and Patterns

By the time your baby reaches the end of the second month, they'll exhibit more deliberate movements, greater physical control, and start developing patterns for eating and sleeping.

- Physical development: Look out for the theatrical appearance of intentional movements. Your baby should be able to turn their head towards sounds and voices, follow objects with their eyes, and hold up their head for longer periods. Around the third month, they might discover their hands and start reaching out for objects.

- Social and emotional development: Between two to four months, babies often begin to reward their parents with smiles. Social smiles are a significant milestone indicating that your baby recognizes the individuals around them.

- Cognitive development: During this period, babies become increasingly alert. They'll start making softer, cooing sounds, experimenting with their vocal cords.

## 8.3. Fifth to the Seventh Month: Recognizing and Interacting

During this period, babies transition from being passive observers to active participants, interacting more with both their surroundings and the people around them.

- Physical development: Your baby's motor skills will improve substantially. By around six months, many babies can roll over in both directions. They also start sitting without support, and some may start crawling around this time.

- Social and Emotional development: This period sees the

development of further social skills like laughing or squealing in delight. Your baby will also identify and mirror the emotions of people around them.

- Cognitive development: Watch out for an explosion in your baby's language progression. From cooing and gurgling, they now start babbling and mimic sounds they hear in their environment. They'll also start understanding and responding to their own name.

# 8.4. Eight to the Twelfth Month: Mastering Motor Skills and Expressing Emotions

The final stretch of the first year is packed with exciting developments, from mastering motor skills to expressing emotions and developing problem-solving abilities.

- Physical development: Expect your baby to master sitting, crawling, standing with support around this time. Manipulating objects, passing them between hands, and using a pincer grip to pick up smaller items become new skills.

- Social and Emotional Development: Babies begin to show signs of separation anxiety and display clear preferences for certain individuals. Look out for expressed enjoyment at games like peek-a-boo as they now understand object permanence.

- Cognitive development: By their first birthdays, most infants can recognize common objects and understand simple instructions paired with gestures.

Understanding your little one's developmental milestones will not only help you support their growth but also be a wonderful way to bond with them and celebrate their journey into becoming individuals. Remember, just as every child is unique, their pace and timing of hitting these milestones can greatly vary. Always consult with your pediatrician if you have any concerns about your baby's development or if they seem to miss any significant milestones. You are about to witness extraordinary growth in your child— enjoy this exhilarating journey!

This concludes one chapter of our comprehensive guide. Following this roadmap closely, you can effectively navigate through the first year of your baby's life, embracing the joys and challenges of parenthood.

# Chapter 9. Selecting the Right Pediatrician

Choosing a pediatrician, one could argue, is one of the first critical judgments we make for our children. This professional will be a key person in your child's life, guiding their health and development from infancy to adolescence. They will also be your consultant, instructor, and confidant in matters of your child's wellbeing. The gravity of this selection calls for a careful, informed and appropriate decision.

## 9.1. The Search for a Pediatrician

Finding prospective pediatricians is as easy as getting referrals from a network of friends, relatives, and healthcare providers. While personal recommendations play an instrumental role, it's also worth doing a quick check online. Pediatrician review sites, local parenting blogs, and local forums can be treasure troves of information.

Remember, every child and every family is unique. What works for one may not work for another. Consider aspects such as the pediatrician's experience, area of expertise, working style, communication skills, and more.

## 9.2. Certification Check

A crucial factor in selecting a pediatrician is their certification. Is the pediatrician board-certified? Board certification indicates that the pediatrician maintains the knowledge, skills, and experience required for the very best pediatric care. This information is often available directly on clinic websites. Reputable clinics will highlight their team's qualification; if this information is not readily available, it could be a cause for concern.

To be more certain, you can visit the official website of the American Board of Pediatrics to confirm a pediatrician's board certification. This additional check serves as a double confirmation and can give peace of mind about your choice.

## 9.3. The First Visit

The first visit to a prospective pediatrician's clinic can be nothing short of an eye-opener. It will even further narrow down your list of the possible options. You get to witness the pediatrician's interaction manner, his/her clinic's surroundings, and other factors that cannot be gleaned from online research or others' experiences.

Observe how the pediatrician interacts with your child, with you, and even, with other patients. Are they patient, kind, understanding, and responsive? A good pediatrician would make your child and you feel comfortable and secure. Interpersonal and communication skills are important markers to take into consideration.

Also, take note of the clinic's cleanliness and modernity of medical equipment. Check the demeanor of the pediatrician's staff and nurses: are they prompt, professional, polite?

## 9.4. Practical Considerations

Practical concerns are equally important as they can influence the pediatrician's availability during short-notice situations. Check the clinic's location: is it accessible from your home, your child's school, or your workplace? Also, check the days and hours of operation: do they align with your availability?

Inquire about their emergency policies: how are off-hour emergencies handled? If the pediatrician is unavailable, is there another board-certified physician who can attend to your child? Also, find out about the typical waiting period for appointments and their policy on taking care of siblings.

# 9.5. Compatibility with Parenting Style and Philosophy

Every parent has unique beliefs concerning their child's upbringing, including approaches to nutrition, immunization, discipline, and more. As such, it's essential to consider a pediatrician whose philosophy aligns with yours.

Discuss these factors with your prospective pediatrician. It's beneficial to clarify things early to prevent clashes in the future. A pediatrician who respects and understands your concerns would be a right fit for you.

# 9.6. Financial Considerations

With the rising costs of healthcare, the financial aspect is an important consideration too. Check if the pediatrician's fees, payment policies, and services covered are within your comfort zone. Does the pediatrician accept your insurance? Are there any extra charges for after-hour services, lengthy discussions, or procedures like vaccinations?

If you are uninsured or have a high deductible, check the pediatrician's policies for self-paying patients. It's better to have these conversations upfront and avoid any unpleasant surprises later.

Choosing the right pediatrician for your child is not a decision to be made overnight. Take your time, perform your due diligence, and trust your instincts. Remember, the best pediatrician for your child is one who makes both of you feel comfortable and cared for. This pediatrician would be a partner in your child's healthcare journey, helping your little one grow into a healthy and happy individual.

Here's to a warm, supportive, and healthy relationship with your chosen pediatrician!

# Chapter 10. Nurturing and Bonding Techniques

Before diving into the myriad ways we can nurture and bond with our newborns, it's important to understand that these techniques should be performed with a heart full of love, patience, consistency, and understanding.

Every baby is unique, and part of the bonding process is getting to know your baby, their preferences, their dislikes, and the subtle cues they give you to communicate. Hence, viewing these techniques as a toolbox from which you can experiment and personalize can be a beneficial approach. So, without further ado, let's step into an enthralling expedition of bonding and supporting the holistic growth of your little one.

## 10.1. The Power of Skin-to-Skin Contact

Skin-to-skin contact or kangaroo care is an extremely effective bonding technique that promotes the physical and emotional well-being of both the parent and the baby.

When a newborn is placed directly onto a parent's bare chest, the baby can hear the parent's heartbeat and breathing, sensations they were familiar with in the womb. This form of contact not only enhances bonding but also stabilizes the baby's heartbeat and temperature, promotes better sleep patterns, reduces crying, and supports breast milk production.

Begin this technique soon after the birth and aim to continue it for as long as both you and the baby find it comforting and beneficial. The touch and closeness are a powerful reassurance of love and safety to your newborn.

## 10.2. Talk, Sing, and Read to Your Baby

Even though your newborn doesn't understand words yet, the soothing sound of your voice does wonders in developing a sense of security and bonding. Plus, it aids in language acquisition much earlier than we might think.

A lullaby before naptime, a gentle chatter during bath time, or a story session can create special bonding moments. It also provides cognitive benefits, building your baby's vocabulary, comprehension, and listening skills even before they start to speak.

## 10.3. Responsive Feeding

Whether breastfeeding or bottle-feeding, each feed is an opportunity to strengthen your bond. Eye contact, skin-to-skin touch, and gentle talk during the feeding time can be profoundly comforting to your baby.

By responding to your baby's cues for hunger and satiety, you imbue them with a sense of being understood and cared for. This responsive feeding approach can contribute to a healthier weight and eating habits as they grow up, along with building trust and attachment.

## 10.4. The Magic of Massage

A gentle baby massage has been a centuries-old tradition across cultures for its numerous benefits. It enhances bonding and helps parents better understand their baby's body language. Also, it stimulates the production of the bonding hormone oxytocin in both the parent and the baby.

Follow a daily or a weekly routine using safe baby oils. Make sure the room is warm enough, your hands are clean, and your movements are gentle but firm. Post-massage, a warm bath can also relax your baby while further promoting your bond.

## 10.5. Babywearing: Closeness On the Go

Babywearing is the practice of carrying your baby in a sling or a carrier. It allows your baby to maintain physical closeness, listen to your heartbeat, feel your warmth, and smell your familiar scent even when you're moving around.

It can be especially beneficial if your baby finds it difficult to settle, as being close to you can soothe them. Plus, it leaves your hands free, which can be a great convenience!

## 10.6. Creating and Sticking To Routines

While they may not seem to appreciate it in the beginning, babies thrive on consistency and routines. Establishing regular patterns for sleeping, feeding, bath time, and play promote a sense of security and predictability in your little one, thereby strengthening your bond.

## 10.7. Mimicking Your Baby

Copy your baby's sounds, gestures, and facial expressions. It might sound silly, but it actually involves engaging in a kind of conversation with your baby. This mirroring behaviour makes them feel important and heard, reinforcing your bond.

Remember, bonding doesn't happen overnight, but with each passing day, your connection grows. Every feed, every nappy change, every smile is a step forward in your beautiful journey of parenthood. Some days might be challenging, but hang in there and know that your love, patience, and commitment are the best gifts for your baby's growth and happiness. As much as these techniques enhance bonding with your newborn, remember that they also facilitate your growth as a parent. So enjoy each moment, and embrace this beautiful phase of life with open arms and an open heart.

# Chapter 11. Surviving and Thriving: Self-Care for New Parents

The journey of being a parent doesn't end with birthing your child; in fact, it's just the beginning. In this phase, you'll learn that self-care is not a luxury you can forego but a necessity for both you and your newborn's health and happiness. The truth is, taking care of a newborn can often feel more than a full-time job. Despite experiencing profound joy, you may also be experiencing fatigue, anxiety, and even depression. Therefore, it's critical to ensure your wellbeing by setting aside time for rest, proper nutrition, exercise, and nurturing creative or personal outlets.

## 11.1. Take Time for Yourself

Taking care of a baby is an almost constant job. Amid diaper changes, feedings, and soothing a crying infant, you may not have a minute left for yourself. But remember, it is not selfish to carve out a pocket of personal time—it's necessary. Even a five-minute break to enjoy a hot cup of tea while your baby is sleeping can serve as a rejuvenating pause. Light exercise, like a walk around the block with your baby in a stroller, can also bring you some well-deserved relaxation. Lean on your support system—be it friends, family, or a babysitter—to watch your baby while you take some time for yourself.

## 11.2. Sleep Enough

The phrase 'sleep when the baby sleeps' could not be truer. Newborns typically sleep 16-18 hours a day, albeit in short stretches. While tempting to rush to complete chores when your baby is sleeping, it's essential to prioritize rest and grab some sleep, as sleep deprivation can have both short and long-term health effects.

## 11.3. Proper Nutrition

Eating healthy meals is a crucial aspect of self-care. What you eat fuels your body, so consuming a balanced diet rich in nutrients, proteins, and good fats will ensure you have the energy needed to provide your baby with the necessary care. Include plenty of fruits, vegetables, and hydration in your diet, especially if you're breastfeeding. If you're finding it difficult to prepare meals, don't hesitate to ask for help or consider meal prepping.

## 11.4. Stay Active

Physical activity can be a fantastic way to promote faster recovery postpartum, help reduce postpartum depression symptoms, and boost your overall mood. Be it light stretching, yoga, or a home workout, ensure you keep it gentle until your doctor gives you a green light for intense activities.

## 11.5. Seek Professional Help

Sometimes, despite all efforts, you may feel overwhelmed, irritable, tired, and unable to cope with daily tasks. These can be signs of postpartum depression. Don't shy away from seeking help. Professional counselors can provide guidance and help you navigate through this journey. Remember, acknowledging that you need help is strength, not weakness.

## 11.6. Connect with Other Parents

It's reassuring to remember that you are not alone. Connecting with other parents can provide solidarity, as they're likely experiencing similar challenges. You can exchange tips, ask for advice, and vent your concerns. Consider joining local parent groups or online forums. These platforms not only foster connections but can also dramatically boost your confidence in your parenthood journey.

## 11.7. Prioritize Emotional Self-Care

Emotional self-care should be a priority. It's okay to feel a myriad of emotions during this period, and it's perfectly acceptable to express them. Parents often experience feelings of anxiety, stress, and frustration. Give yourself permission to escape the constant hum of baby care tasks by investing time in activities you love, like reading a book, painting, or even gardening.

## 11.8. Partner Cooperation

Raising a child is a collective responsibility, especially if you have a partner. Both should share baby-related tasks, supporting each other both emotionally and physically. Open communication can help balance the workload and ensure that both people's needs are met, making the journey smoother and happier.

In conclusion, self-care is pivotal in your transition into parenthood. It's not selfish but crucial - for you and your newborn. Armed with these self-care tips, you're well-equipped to tackle the challenges that come your way while taking care of your newborn. Remember, it's okay to take a step back, breathe, and care for yourself. You deserve it!

9 7 9 8 8 5 6 2 6 2 5 1 2